T0129629

THE HANDBOOK OF SEXUALITY:

A Semi-Humorous Guide to Human Sexuality

DR. P.Y. SUN

BALBOA
PRESS

A DIVISION OF HAY HOUSE

Balboa Press books may be ordered through booksellers or by contacting:

Balboa Press
A Division of Hay House
1663 Liberty Drive
Bloomington, IN 47403
www.balboapress.com
1 (877) 407-4847

Print information available on the last page.

ISBN: 978-1-9822-2693-0 (sc)
ISBN: 978-1-9822-2700-5 (e)

Library of Congress Control Number: 2019905038

Balboa Press rev. date: 08/19/2019

CONTENTS

DEDICATION

To my parents, Peter and Vera Sun, without whom I would not be here.

I. WHAT WENT WRONG

CHAPTER 1

Introduction

I remember in medical school being made to watch a film of a man's hand masturbating his penis to erection. Then the film talked about erectile latency. This is not what Sexuality is about.

Sexuality is the way we communicate

our need for relationships, or at least flirting ☺ I call the book a Handbook because it is organized with sections under the headings of the common sexual descriptions –the Slut, the Prude, etc…

CHAPTER 2

The Slut, with subsection Skanks

A butt in my face. A <u>woman</u>'s. At a coffeehouse. UGH.

Sluts will use their body inappropriately for the meanest reasons –such as above for *crazy* attention. My idea of a slut is someone who sleeps with a man she isn't even attracted to (or a man with a woman, in these times of increasing number of gigolos) –to get concert tickets, worth about $20-30.

Another example is the slut who brushed her breast against **my** breasts at a restaurant. Was she advertising that she could be bought for a cheap price?

The classic example of a slut is someone, usually a woman, who wears a low-cut shirt + short skirt + very tight clothes + lots of makeup + overworked hair + absurdly high heels. It describes the woman who caught a rich Persian that I knew.

Surprisingly, she also had a brain –but you really had to focus past all that in-your-face advertising. In this case, the man had poor taste and did not understand that by being with that woman, men with worth wrote him off as low-class. She is not an example of a classic slut, as she was successful in getting a well-to-do man. That is more like a prostitute of this day and age (see next chapter). However, her dress fit exactly the image of a slut.

Which begs the question –is it beneficial to be a slut? Back in cave man days when many children were lost to a dangerous environment, it may have been. Now, we just have easy people –easy to fertilize/ aggressive inseminators, with probably poor character traits. I used to think a lack of taste was not too important –per popular wisdom; however, I now know that poor taste is a type of delusion. Not to be taken lightly!

Being popular is over-rated. Thus, we have someone dressing like a slut and being rewarded with more than $20-30 for it.

It's almost like the shifting of adulthood from the teenage years to one's 30's that we see these days, when in fact puberty is hitting people even earlier than in the 1800's –probably because of increased hormones in our food.

Will skanks become the norm for what

people should be in the next generation? Which brings us to ask what is the definition of a skank? Perhaps an example is best:

One woman, just to annoy me, straddled her legs around me –kinda like a Basic Instinct movie move. How low can you go???

You see lots of skanks in trailer parks –once again, all the characteristic dress of a slut, with just the aim to annoy or irritate by using their bodies.

They will take off their tops to fluster a man. A male skank will moon someone. One day, I was driving on the California freeway, and a young man in the passenger seat *mooned* me while I was driving. It upset me immensely —however, being a good driver, I just got away from him. I wonder if he had mooned an inadequate driver if he would have caused a 10-car pileup?

CHAPTER 3

The Prostitute

Carrie's friend from *Sex in the City*, Samantha. A publicity businesswoman. Lives in a swank rent-control. The only drawback being the older women who looked down their noses at her because she earned her own pull and money instead of inheriting it from a husband or father.

Most men are prostitutes –meaning they use their body wrongly to obtain money. The old-fashioned way was to be a workaholic or a quasi-gigolo. Nowadays, one sees a mix of the two modes, almost indiscriminately.

As a definition, a prostitute –whose work is worth perhaps $20-$30/ hour, is paid $200-$300/ hour as a prostitute, paralleling the ones who walk the street to sell sex instead of having a secretarial job.

The highest paid positions are usually prostitutes. Thus, the doctor is only in the upper-middle earning sector. The wrong those prostitutes commit *seems* less toxic than physical misdemeanors/ felonies –lying with their mouths, spending time with people they really dislike, and contorting their body to make it seem like they like their clients. Some are exceptional actors. Perhaps they don't have the looks to be a multi-million-dollar salary actor, but they have the charm to eventually make it to the million-dollar stage. Their sexuality is used on both men and women, whatever the prostitute's gender. To the same gender, they are BFFs "best friends forever." To the opposite gender, they are the quintessential admirer.

The prostitute also usually has a very

recognizable wardrobe. Perhaps not the (1) low-cut shirt + (2) short skirt + (3) very tight clothes + (4) lots of makeup + (5) overworked hair + (6) absurdly high heels of a slut, but a limited combination of the above –say, (1) + (3) +(6) or (2) + (3) + (4) + (5). Carrie's friend in *Sex in the City* –she wore sexy clothes for brunch that should have been reserved for a nighttime outing at a club.

The desperate housewives of lore would also lure men (milkmen, mailmen) who came by their lonely houses with a slip of the robe, walking naked by a window... How many children were inseminated by the gardener or pool boy? Was the husband secretly happy that he had a son even if not of his own blood because his "soldiers" weren't getting the job done? The mixing of the gene pool puts the "blue-blood" theory to naught.

With prostitutes, it is difficult to say who the parents of a child are. Housewives often marry a man who has enough money to provide a house –left to the housewife when he dies or when they divorce, the latter being more common. The prostitutes are often not interested in or adept at being parents. Thus, family members or others in the community become the caregivers. At times, it is a result of drug addiction that someone is unable to parent.

The close relationship between addiction and prostitution is well known. They say that pimps get the prostitute hooked on drugs to better control the prostitute. I think it also works the other way —where the loss of a soul and the pain of selling oneself leads the prostitute to seek relief in drugs.

In the case of Samantha, she seemed to seek relief in great sex. I find it funny that when a young, successful, hot actor wanted to settle down with her, she could not make the step to settling down. Perhaps something got broken when she misused her body for so long. The human being is made to be whole, to have integrity. When you separate the soul and emotions from the body, there comes a point of *no return*. **The superficiality becomes permanent.**

CHAPTER 4

The Prude

Speaking of Desperate Housewives, we now move one to the example of Bree of Wisteria Lane. Bree, the prude, also separated her sexuality from the rest of her soul.

Bree was the ultimate housewife—excellent cook, tidy housekeeper, not so satisfying in bed. Her husband was a medical doctor who went to a dominatrix to feel satisfied. We'll talk about the dominatrix part later.

In fact, Bree was the dominant figure in the household, so the need to be dominated shared by some men was inherent in her husband's messed-up psychology. She just wasn't adventurous in bed.

Later on, Bree gets involved with a lesser medical professional, and then finally someone who understands her. She evolved past the targeting of the housewife's "perfect husband."

Usually women do not peak in their sexuality until they are able to shed the brainwashing of their youth, sometime in their 40's –when they begin to enjoy sex. (I am talking about women who are now in at least their thirties' génération.)

It is not just women who succumb to a society's illnesses about sexuality. I know a boy-man, well in his 30's, who tried to please women from a restricted society by rubbing his penis against their pelvis, but not penetrating. Servicing the technical virgins.

It took him about 10 times longer than the normal way to ejaculate, but the girl's contacts I guess were worth pleasing and keeping the technical virgin serviced.

I have heard of some couples that are technical virgins after dating for more than 2 years, but in the process mess up their sexualities. How is it healthier to use only one's hands and mouths in sex? Perhaps in terms of genital diseases (although there is often rubbing of the genitals involved), but this couple was religious and was doing it for their conscious. Yet oral sex is still sex! And less satisfying if one is in an intimate relationship.

I would equate it to the bitches that won't use the word "fuck," but fuck everyone in sight with their meanness or cruelty.

Technical word virgins. Not something to emulate.

Now back to the issue of a dominatrix. They are just the other side of the coin, the complement (no not a compl*i*ment) of the illness of the prude. A prude needs someone to push past their inhibition in sexuality, and a dominatrix is the most convenient societal service for men to get past their inhibitions –the yang to their yin (just kidding, those terms are used in a compl*i*mentary way). Men are into convenience, and unfortunately –less so into health.

You can find women with a healthy

sexuality to bring the man from prudeness to being sexually healthy, better than into another form of illness as with the dominatrix. The sexually healthy woman is rarer and probably has a much higher price attached in terms of effort, time, and other resources in order to court her. In the end, the healthy woman is harder to persuade to accept an unhealthy man than a dominatrix.

CHAPTER 5

The Frigid, with subsection Sexual Dysfunction

No amount of tying up, studs, or whips can warm up the frigid. I have no stories of dating frigids, thank God.

It is even a category in Sexual Dysfunctions in mental health. How would it feel like to have never experienced an orgasm? Physiologically, the human being functions with occasional to consistent sexual satisfaction. We are even programmed to be able to arouse ourselves, usually with the help of some mental images or emotions.

The frigid cannot overcome their brainwashing; while the prude has hope. Who knows what trauma they experienced, whether rape or the slow drip of being told one is not *worthy* if one is sexual.

Many men brought up in the same society as a frigid woman will prefer a frigid for a "wife." Then, they know that the woman won't be turned on by the milkman or the mailman. These men seek sexual fulfillment outside the house.

Other than that, there is no place for the frigid.

Sexual dysfunction can take many forms. For a man, many times it is erectile dysfunction. Anxiety seems to me to be a large proportionate cause of this category. Performance anxiety is often joked about, but even specific anxiety of *other* topics can affect function. For example, perhaps they are close to getting fired. In terms of sexuality, they are blocked by their anxiety and are not able to exude the healthy energy that is sexuality. They radiate the unhealthy energy of anxiety instead.

Funny enough, many people have SEX to relieve some anxiety. That is, before the anxiety becomes pathological and they have a recognized mental illness.

Another common cause of sexual dysfunction is medication. Impotency is as bad as it sounds. Other medications cause decreased libido, or sexual desire.

Some of these people seem a little genderless. You can stand beside them at a nudist colony, and you feel no sexuality from them. No flirtation, no desire for attention that is sexually-charged.

Some people seem born that way, kinda the opposite of a hermaphrodite, someone who has both sexual organs. A lot of sexuality does come from the hormones produced by the sexual organs. Pheromones are the scent-laden secretions of sexuality. In animals, they can be detected MILES away.

Some people have somewhat repulsive pheromones. They also secrete any chemical imbalance or medication they are on. Most men seem able to overcome visual, audio, or olfactory repulsion if they are horny enough. Women usually are more selective, unless they are a skank or slut. However, in this society of encouraging sluts, the proportion of garbage in the population has doubled. Be careful when dating (our next chapter), there are very few quality people available.

Thus, ends Section I: What Went Wrong.

II. WHAT IS WORTHWHILE

What is Worthwhile. Read on.

▐▌

CHAPTER 6

Dating

At a coffeehouse. A blonde WOMAN's butt in my face (I am a healthy heterosexual woman). Not what I was looking for –hook-up or not, at a coffeehouse.

I once went to a coffeehouse that had the neat idea of being a dating spot. Public, safe place to meet for a first date. People hung up notecards about themselves and who they were looking for. For me, it was a little too anti-septic, a little too safe.

Romance is exhilarating. At least in the way that embodies its essence. We date for affection and attention. There is nothing like that special someone looking at you, looking deeply or even covertly into each other's eyes.

Infatuation sets in –if we're lucky. Deep sighs. That's longing.

For some, the longing stops in the groins. For others, it reaches the heart.

How long does the infatuation last?

Two-six months seems the average, depending on the amount of tantalizing self-denial.

For example, there were some knights of King Arthur who never touched Guinevere, yet probably longed chastely for years (if we don't count masturbation).

Chaste and anti-septic are not synonyms. The knights burned with passion for her. Danger accompanied the knights' missions for the queen. They transferred their passion for the woman to a passion for their missions. Their infatuation lasted probably longer than 6 months.

During the infatuation phase –let's say

6 months for modern day's sake, one can get to know each other as whole persons, or just focus on the physical. Oftentimes, I find that the latter couple fizzle out by 6 months' time, not even time usually to get engaged –luckily.

One guy I know said his "relationships" always fizzled out sexually by 1 year, no matter how sex-starved he was. I also noticed he showed no inclination to get to know a woman –or make an effort emotionally.

Men seem to know who they want to be with within a month. Some tell me they know who they want to *marry* <u>within a month</u>! I don't know if it's because men expect less or that they are simpler in their desires. Perhaps both.

How much has nature programmed the woman to be the pacer of a romantic relationship? For myself, I always trusted a guy to lead —which got me into lots of trouble. I do believe that some men <u>are</u> more gifted in being the pacemaker, perhaps they are the real catches.

It used to be that the only reason for dating was to figure out whether the man and woman were compatible for marriage. I am one of those old-fashionedly brought-up people.

Then again, dating can be an end to

itself. It is enough of a vehicle for physical satisfaction, including sex.

It is enough of a vehicle for the traditional business-oriented union. He needs her father's contacts or a place to stay and she wants the legitimacy of having an escort. Many places still look down on a woman attending functions by herself, whether business or social.

Is it enough to have companionship in dating, i.e. without the sex? Probably not. Therein lies the rub. The most undervalued benefit of a being a couple is also the most overlooked in modern dating.

CHAPTER 7

The Sexy, the Hot, and the Romantic

If we are lucky, we will date one of the above.

Picture, if you are a guy, dating Eva Longoria or a Sophia Loren. Or if you are a woman —sexy Brad Pitt or Roger Moore. They exude that "je ne sais quoi" or hard-to-define essence that is sexiness. However hard as it may be to focus on the *other* dimensions of a relationship when dating someone like them, it is always good flirting.

Picture Megan Fox or a Taylor Lautner. Now we are getting to the Hot. What is the difference between Hot and Sexy? Someone once said that it is the mind that is Sexy. So it goes to reason that the body is what makes someone Hot (without necessarily the qualities of a higher mind). A Sophia Loren could have been a medical doctor, but a Megan Fox can be a mechanic. (Actually, Megan Fox seems smart enough to be a modern-day doctor, now that it has become mostly technical skills). The two professions are very close in skills, but a higher talent in art and a higher call to professionalism is required for the former.

Sexiness is hard to find, especially in the traditional woman who is raised to <u>not</u> value, and at times underplay, her mind. So, most men settle for a *hot* woman. Then again, the men who do <u>not</u> possess the higher qualities in the mind *themselves* do not appreciate the sexiness of an intelligent woman. How then do intelligent women attract not-so-intelligent men (or vice-versa in this age of accepted aggressive women)? The bridge between would be the Romantic, who utilizes the tantalizing effects of romance to paint the loveliest picture possible of his or her lover.

Ah –the Romantic. I mentioned the exhilaration of romance and King Arthur's round table in the previous chapter. For some unknown, probably chemical reason –romance kick-starts the fireworks that communicate sexual love or romantic love. Love at first sight is probably based mostly on these chemical reactions, including pheromones and hormones. Myself, I like to believe that it is also based on past experiences and one's judgement if one is quick enough to love at first sight (versus infatuation or horniness).

I have been struck by this lightning twice in my lifetime, and I consider myself lucky even though they both didn't work out. For me, this meant unsuccessful dating that didn't end in marriage. The second time didn't even involve sexual interactions, i.e. not even a kiss!

Recently, I felt a strong pull that wasn't love at first sight, but definitely infatuation at first sight. The man I met right away jump-started the romantic juices. He spontaneously declared a poem to me, exclaiming "that face!" which led me to be suspicious that he had used the poem before. He hadn't. The infatuation ripened so that I actually thought he was more and more handsome.

I took the time to get to know him and found out that he had wild mood swings and an unrealistic view of romance. That level of romance can lead to the "what went wrong" path instead of the "what is worthwhile" road. For example, the same man talked about "an angel" falling from heaven (a woman) and he fell and hit his eye on the corner of the pavement. Oww!

CHAPTER 8

The Modest and
the Natural

What do you think of when you think
of someone modest? Someone who is
above average but *says* they are "average"?
Actually, that is a good description of being
humble –a characteristic that I think is
over-rated –being a more natural person

myself. Humbleness seems to be a societal nicety at best, a means of manipulation to be able better to take advantage of others at worst.

Anyway, a modest person can be, say, above average –but she doesn't tell it to the mountains. That is, she is not boastful –which seems to be the opposite of being humble as we see in modern society. In declaring that they are "*so low*," they are announcing themselves far and wide.

Being natural is like being romantic; too much can also be a problem. In the natural world, testosterone is king in the male species –so much so that many times animals die unnecessarily because of their hormones. On the female side, I've watched my cat EAT her newborn. Maybe it was sick or maybe it was stillborn, I don't know. Perhaps it is one way of getting nutrition in the natural world, when an animal is dead or sickly. But what I do know is that we don't cotton to that as humans. An amount of self-restraint is necessary, even if one is natural.

I believe that it is the self-restraint of modesty that makes it a positive attribute of sexuality without the negative –negative like being hot or sexy *without* having self-restraint. One may have *other* negative traits while being hot, like being simplistic, but that is not intrinsic to being hot –although it seems to be prevalent when one is lacking refinement of mind.

Besides being confused with humbleness, I think that modesty is confused with a self-deprecatory tendency. Again, it fits the example of humbleness above with the "*so low* comment, but the self-deprecation is more encompassing and compulsive. It is a learned behavior, especially for women and certain cultures.

Natural is what it sounds –encompassing the beneficial attributes of sexuality: powerful, necessary, and beneficial. The negative tendencies of being natural: destructive, overly-aggressive, laziness can be seen when one is natural without being mindful, i.e. without Freud's superego or one's conscious. The conscious is part of being natural —and I believe animals also have a superego, if more limited.

But in being human, a more complex superego is required –thus, we don't condone mothers to eat their sickly newborns. We demand that men don't duel to the death anymore over a dame. We ask that people don't leave potholes in the street, even if the natural tendency for an animal would be to leave the pothole if oneself knows where it is, and those one cares for knows. Strangers be damned.

Yet not only do we demand that potholes not exist in society, look at the commercial from Domino's Pizza that advertises what I consider a rather unrelated topic of fixing potholes so that the consumer buys their pizzas. We ask that the general public call and tell others about the potholes. That is the morality and ethics that I learned growing up.

CHAPTER 9

Sex

What is wrong with a one-night stand? Society says it is wrong. With sexuality, it may not be so.

A friend of mine told me about what she once did on St. Patrick's Day. She had been invited by a friend to a luncheon where she did not know anybody else. There was a tall, semi-attractive American —talking about his big penis, hitting on her there. But it was the European who caught her eye. At least 10 years older than the American, but with more substance. His mentee, about 20 years younger, also was making a move —but he had an off-putting egocentricity. The attractive bartender woman was *herself* hitting on the older European.

They decided to get out of the luncheon, my friend and the older European. He said they should stop and get dinner (many hours had passed by then and it was about time for the next meal). A good sign, she said to herself. Yet at dinner, all he talked about in a crass way was sex.

By the time they reached his hotel –he was on one of his frequent business trips, it was late enough for her to feel the effects of eating all day and the champagne. As she lay in bed, he got on top of her and did the deed. None of the highly-charged, sexy moves he did even while driving his car. Then, later in the night, he did it again.

In the morning, he was quiet, but expectant. She didn't ask for his number. He made a move to get her number, but she did not encourage him. He looked confused.

She chalked it up to an experiment.

The European had explained that he had just gotten out of a 3-year relationship that included 2 children, and how his girlfriend had "changed" after having the first child. It seemed he was relieved that he was able to be comfortable around another woman.

My friend was non-plussed to be the replacement "comfortable' girl. She was looking for sexy and romantic, which was what he exuded at the restaurant. A successful, family-business man, he exuded a kind of confidence that was sexy to all the women –including the pretty bartender!

How disappointing was his "phone-it-in" sex, in contrast.

Here was an example how the teaser of sexuality did not deliver at sex.

In the opposite manner, I last dated a man with whom I had the best sex of my life, as the time of this writing in April of 2017. However, his everyday behavior –even at a restaurant where good, sensual food was being served, was lackluster.

Being old-fashioned, I don't believe sex to be the most important component of a relationship –especially if one wishes to remain a couple as one gets elderly. The sex kept the relationship going for months longer than it should have. He related a similar experience he had had where he wasn't even dating the woman but kept getting together with her. There was a surly despair in his demeanor that came from not having the capacity to reason through relationships or talk to the woman he is dating.

Sex. One reason why some have a strong sexuality. The European and the –let's call him Mr. Surly, radiated sexuality. Mr. Surly delivered in bed, the European did not. Yet both struck out for the women who want a relationship –not just flirting, sex, or a "phone-it-in" mentality! They may fill in the gap for women who just want to become pregnant, or deliver one's seed if one is a man. Either gender not wanting a relationship. Thus, the redemption of the one-night stand.

I did date someone who put my first, an American lover, to shame in the bedroom. He also wanted a relationship and children (being French dictated the latter). But he had a melancholy that was overpowering, even thought we shared the joys of food, sex, and intellectualism.

Sex cannot overcome the basic serious flaws in a relationship. It can become divorced from a relationship, hence the "friends with benefits" category that has become popular these days. Again, an unhealthy popularity.

The glue that holds a relationship together was missing in the 2 men of the first examples: Mr. Surly and the European (ok let's call it as it is, the Dutch). Sexual love, or Eros, is the flypaper that makes the relationship an exclusive love. (More about love in the next chapter.) When it's just sex, it can be found in non-relationships. Perhaps not as good as the primary lover, but good enough if one is impatient to wait for when your lover is in the mood, or on geographical trips.

The Dutch's ex-girlfriend may have been ok with the stability of having a successful man who gives money for children, but is not faithful. No one in Mr. Surly's past was a girlfriend for long, after his college days. He seemed stuck on his romantic failures, and was no longer able to sustain even a purely sexual liaison.

After sex should come love. Men seem to often function this way. It can happen the other way –with love coming before sex, which occurs with most women and men who are thoughtful and self-controlled; but biologically speaking (as it takes two to tango) ...

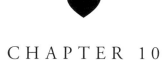

Love

Sexual love, or the "Eros" as the Greek defined it, is a love in which one constantly longs to be with that one person. No one else will do. Even in groups, one is lonely without that person. How long sexual love lasts seems variable. Do not confuse lust for sexual love. Lust seems to last just a couple of months.

Is two years —the "honeymoon" period, a better indicator of the lasting power of sexual love? What about the golden anniversary-celebrating couple who truly are still in love with each other after 50 years?? Is being "in love" the same as sexual love? Is it a **voluntary** love, as some have tried to define love, or a purely a chemical reaction?

I would venture to say that sexual love and being "in love" are different. Many times, lust may be a sub-category of being "in love" and is more short-term. Sexual love seems a more intermediate love, between being "in love" and intimacy or friendship. Of course, friendship can also be short-lived, but usually one hallmark of friendship is the it stands the test of time.

Perhaps sexual love is that "glue" that allows a couple to navigate the waters between being "in love" and intimacy.

A couple of months is not enough for most (women) to know if one wants to spend "the rest of one's life" with someone. Sexual love seems to last about 1 year, according to the example in the last chapter of the man who had only sexual interest in a woman for 1 year, because he did not desire a real emotional connection. However, if one has <u>some</u> emotional connection, the "honeymoon" period of 2 years applies.

Now, for the couple that seems to still be "newlyweds" in their 60's, a less than 1% of couples –what is their secret? They seem to renew their emotional/ spiritual bond regularly. Of course, they have the capacity for long-term relationship as well. They understand the human need for companionship that goes along with a relationship.

The most lasting ingredient is spiritual love. That is often called agape, or "unconditional" love. The best example is the love of a parent for her child.

Many times, I find the <u>man</u> treats the woman like a child. I guess that may make the relationship last longer, but I'd like to be living in reality as well. The best solution for me is to be a "girl-woman" and for my partner to be a "boy-man." I have always preferred this type of man to date –maybe I wasn't wrong.

Now, to the question of whether loving is voluntary. I believe that I have shown that the long-term love is achieved with effort –the effort to work at a relationship instead of relying solely on chemical reactions within our brain. For those elderly couples who achieve love without sex —it is the replaying of the ideal love of medieval times that comprises a "chaste" love.

Yet the elderly couple is smarter in being able to also tap into the potential of companionship that is built-into a real relationship. In addition to the friendship, the long-term couple has the romance that is the whipped cream that makes almost anything sweet even better.

To have a lasting, romantic relationship is the goal of anyone who is healthy. #

#Even monks and nuns express their love, including their romantic need for love, to God. Have you ever read their writings? Some of their writings would make erotica seem tame ☺

WARNING TO READER

I hope the reader finds this manual helpful and humorous in their own journey of sexuality. Sexuality has many misconceptions, the first being that it is only about sex.

This book is an attempt at being informative and amusing. As an analogy, it asks questions akin to, "Why are people called blue-blood?" Is it the unoxygenated hemoglobin? How about having a "yellow" tint? Unbroken-down bilirubin —with Mediterranean green tint being a mixture? Okay, **The handbook of Sexuality** is less technical and more sensational. Enjoy!

ACKNOWLEDGEMENTS

I would like to thank the people who believe in my writing and the wisdom of being healthy: my benefactors, mentors, and readers! I am lucky in having people who support my work without having to be mentioned by name.

I am grateful to Hay House for their belief in my work, and their quick responses to my questions. Thanks to Melanie Foursha for taking the time to get me on board.

I am thankful for the people who continue to ensure that Medicine will be centered around the patient/ client, and will not be based solely on greed, fear, or a desire for influence. Please read my first book: The TRUE Face of Health Care Reform: A Physician and Patient's Perspective for the discussion on what is needed in health care.

Printed in the United States
By Bookmasters